BILLY, ME & YOU

Nicola Streeten

BILLY, ME & YOU

A MEMOIR OF GRIEF AND RECOVERY

First published in 2011 by

Myriad Editions
59 Lansdowne Place
Brighton BN3 1FL, UK

www.MyriadEditions.com

1 3 5 7 9 10 8 6 4 2

A CIP catalogue record for this book is available from
the British Library.

ISBN: 978-0-9565599-4-4

Printed in China on paper sourced from sustainable forests.

For John and Sally

PART ONE

Wed Thu Fri Sat Sun | Mon Tue Wed Thu Fri Sat Sun | Mon Tue Wed Thu Fri Sat Sun | Mon Tue Wed Thu Fri Sat Sun | Mon Tue Wed

2 3 4 5 6 7 8 9 10 11 12 13 14 15 16 17 18 19 20 21 22 23 24 25 26 27 28 29 30 31

I HAD HELD BACK MY TEARS AT
THE HOSPITAL. RIDICULOUS, BUT
I HADN'T WANTED TO FURTHER
UPSET OUR FAMILIES. BACK
HOME, IT FELT SAFE TO
RELEASE MY EMOTIONS.

THE CRYING THING WAS SO
STRANGE. I CRIED EVERY DAY
FOR A YEAR AFTER BILLY
DIED, BUT ONLY EVER IN FRONT
OF JOHN OR THE PSYCHOLOGIST.
...NOT EVEN IN FRONT OF
MY MOTHER... NOT EVEN
AT THE FUNERAL.

THIS DAILY CRYING WAS A
PSYCHOLOGICAL NECESSITY,
LIKE A BOWEL MOVEMENT.

BUT I WAS TERRIFIED BY
THE SURROUNDING TABOO
—THE SOCIAL LIMITS TO
THE DISPLAY OF GRIEF
AND THE INVOLUNTARY
JUDGEMENTS OF OTHERS.

AT THE SAME TIME I KNEW
I WOULD LOSE MY MIND IF I
BOTTLED UP SUCH INTENSE PAIN.

I KNEW THAT TALKING ABOUT IT WAS ALLOWED — POSITIVELY ENCOURAGED, WITHIN THE LIBERAL CIRCLES IN WHICH I MIXED.

THE MORE I TOLD PEOPLE, THE MORE INTRIGUED I BECAME AT THEIR RESPONSES... I FOUND MYSELF JUDGING PEOPLE BY THEIR REACTIONS.

THE MOST COMMON RESPONSE WAS FOR PEOPLE, EVEN STRANGERS, TO GET WATERY-EYED. THIS FASCINATED ME THE MOST… DID THEY GET THAT EVERY TIME THEY WATCHED STORIES OF DEAD CHILDREN ON THE NEWS?

THE WINNING REPLIES WERE FROM TWO OF MY STUDENTS, HAKIMA AND KARIM, IN SPITE OF THEIR LIMITED ENGLISH.

BUT ON THE DAY BILLY DIED, I STILL HAD A LONG JOURNEY AHEAD.

19 9 '95

LATER, DON AND MEL BROUGHT THE
CAR BACK AND STAYED FOR A CUP
OF TEA· MEL MOVED BILLY'S TOP OUT
OF THE WAY AS SHE SAT DOWN·

SO THIS WAS GRIEF. A THING WITH A LIFE OF ITS OWN — CONTROLLING AND DISTORTING OUR UNDERSTANDING OF THE WORLD — TURNING THE INNOCENT GESTURES OF KIND PEOPLE WHO LOVED US INTO MALICIOUS ACTS OF SPITE.

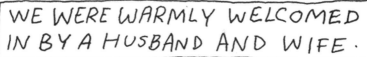

WE WERE WARMLY WELCOMED IN BY A HUSBAND AND WIFE.

TEA?

YES, PLEASE

IT WAS AN UTTERLY PERFECT CUP OF TEA ··· WITH THE CORRECT BISCUITS.

SINCE BILLY DIED I'D BEEN OBSESSING ABOUT TOP-SHELF BISCUITS (BISCUIT PORN?) YOU KNOW THE KIND... OVERPRICED, CONTINENTAL, QUALITY CHOCOLATE, HARDLY ANY IN A PACKET, SERVED WITH GOOD TEA.

SO THE MAIN THINGS IN MY LIFE HAD SPIRALLED OUT OF CONTROL BUT A COMFORTING ORDER COULD BE CREATED THROUGH THE DETAIL. SHE KNEW THAT—THIS WOMAN WHO LOST HER BABY SIX YEARS AGO.

AFTER SHE DIED WE GOT RID OF EVERYTHING TO DO WITH HER... I REGRET THAT SO MUCH...

THE FORMAT WAS SIMILAR TO A MOTHER AND BABY GROUP WHERE YOU SWAP BIRTH STORIES AND EXCHANGE TIPS FOR COPING WITH YOUR NEW STATUS.

I TARMACKED OVER THE FRONT GARDEN

SOME WEEKS LATER WE ATTENDED
A GROUP AT THE HOSPITAL RUN BY
A FRIENDLY NURSE. IT WAS OUR FIRST
VISIT BACK TO THE HOSPITAL.

My daughter died at one day old. I got pregnant again straight away. This time I had a boy and he is fine, but all I can think about is my little girl that I lost. My husband refuses to speak about her.

our baby girl died at two days old. Then we had another baby... ...Also a girl...she died when she was four days old...

The tests I had during my pregnancy showed very severe deformities in my baby. I decided to have a termination and because my pregnancy was ... advanced ... I had to give birth ... and ... when my son was delivered ... 0 .. 00 .. he had .. 0 .. no deformities ...

My son was born with a number of heart abnormalities. He spent a lot of his life here in the hospital and died when he was eight.

THEN...IT WAS OUR TURN

AND THEN, FROM THIS INTENSE SHARING OF PAIN AND TEARS, THE MOOD CHANGED TO ONE OF HILARITY. OUR FOCUS TURNED TO THE COMIC ASPECTS OF OUR EXPERIENCES.

ha ha ha ha

We talked about having headstones and ashes in our living rooms while we decided what to do with them ... and forgetting they were there ...

ha ha

ha ha

ha ha

... and people's confusion if they saw them and

DIDN'T KNOW

hee hee

... and how often people who DIDN'T KNOW would make

OH

hee hee

YES

"*that face*"

AT THE END, I ASKED THE PSYCHOLOGIST WHAT SHE'D THOUGHT OF THE MEETING.

IT WASN'T WHAT I'D EXPECTED

EVER SINCE, I HAVE WONDERED WHAT SHE **HAD** EXPECTED.

THE WORST MEETING WE ATTENDED WAS AT A DIFFERENT HOSPITAL. IT WAS SOME SORT OF NATIONAL MEETING OF BEREAVED PARENTS... WE ALL HAD DEAD CHILDREN... NOTHING WOULD BRING THEM BACK... THE FORMAT WAS THE SAME... WE TOLD OUR STORIES...

ONE WOMAN'S EMOTION FILLED THE PLACE... WE ARE SUING THE HOSPITAL The Surgeon was negligent and shows NO sense of REMOR or responsibility

ANGER INJUSTICE BLAME

HER STORY THREATENED
THE BASIC PREMISE OF
MY "SOFT ZONE" WHICH
WAS THAT PEOPLE ARE
HONEST, KIND AND
HELPFUL ... YES, OF
COURSE I WAS BLOCKING
STUFF OUT, BUT ...

my soft zone

.. IF MY SOFT ZONE GOT DAMAGED I KNEW KILLING MYSELF WOULD HAVE TOO MUCH APPEAL

That's why I had to leave that meeting

MEANWHILE I CARRIED ON DOING MY JOB TEACHING NIGHT CLASSES · BUT MY WALK HOME WAS BECOMING INCREASINGLY DIFFICULT·

JOHN HAD FELT UNABLE TO RETURN TO HIS WORK OR STUDIO·

HE'D STARTED TO SPEND MORE AND MORE TIME IN BED...

THAT NIGHT I DREAMED...

I CONTINUED TO TALK OPENLY TO FRIENDS ABOUT MY EXPERIENCE, SO I SUPPOSE I SHOULDN'T HAVE BEEN SURPRISED BY **THEM** TALKING OPENLY TO ME ABOUT MY EXPERIENCE ... BUT SOMETIMES I WAS...

SO WHEN I STARTED TO SEE "MY" THERAPIST, I HAD PLENTY TO UNLOAD.

IT MUST BE RETRIBUTION
FOR MY SMUGNESS AND
FOR NOT SEEING HOW
LUCKY I WAS.

PUNISHMENT
FROM A GOD I
DON'T BELIEVE IN.

HAD I BEEN A BAD PARENT? WAS THAT IT?

I REMEMBERED HOW MY LIFE HAD BEEN.

WE LIVED AT 40 b

OUR FRIEND 'DIGGIE' LIVED AT 40 a

DOWNSTAIRS WAS AN EMPTY SHOP

KEBABS

40

OUR LANDLORD WAS KIND AND FAIR. HE GOT DEPRESSION AND OFTEN SKIPPED HIS MEDICATION BECAUSE IT NUMBED HIM TOO MUCH.

HE DECIDED TO TURN THE EMPTY SHOP DOWNSTAIRS INTO A CHARITY SHOP.

ON HIS GOOD DAYS HE ENJOYED DRESSING UP IN THE DONATED CLOTHES.

THE TOP OF THE MORNING TO YOU

FOR ALL CHARITIES:-
THE DEAF
THE DUMB
THE HANDICAPPED

SUDDENLY HE WENT TO VISIT FAMILY IN IRELAND AND NEVER RETURNED.

The Calling of St Anthony

Integrity
Dignity
Humour
Teeth
Hair
Heart
Love
Temper
Grip
Life
Vision
Souls
Kidneys
Eyes
Limbs
Mind
Sight
Truth
Fortune
Faith
Friendship
Health
Home
Confidence
Taste
Smell
Way
Strength
Skill
Passion
Honour
White cells
Red cells
Self respect
Magic
Cool
Marbles
etc. etc.

The patron saint of all things lost

THEY WERE SELLING THEIR WORKS FOR JUST A FEW POUNDS. WE BOUGHT THIS TEXT PIECE BY TRACEY EMIN.

THE NEXT TIME I CAME ACROSS THAT ARTWORK WAS ON THE DAY BILLY DIED.

I arrived home with a splitting headache...

... why do some people say they've "lost" someone...

when they mean that person is DEAD?

IT WASN'T JUST THE JOURNAL. WE HAD CREATED AN ARCHIVE OF OBJECTS AND WRITINGS. LATER THESE BECAME PROMPTS FOR THE TELLING OF OUR STORY.

LOOK! BILLY'S LAST CRISP PACKET, WITH SOME CRISPS STILL IN IT

EUGH! PRESERVED MOULD

A favourite bib

Billy's milk bottle, melted down in a forgotten sterilising process

My successful pregnancy test

My journals

I'D FORGOTTEN HIS CONFUSION OVER OUR NON-RELIGIOUS WISHES.

AND HIS ASSUMPTION THAT BILLY HADN'T COUNTED
IN OUR LIVES QUITE SO MUCH, BEING "JUST A BABY"

Private Lives

Next problem

Your baby girl seemed perfect when she was born – but she died at just three days old. How can you come to terms with your loss?

Lesbian, Gay and
...ety. It featured photos
..., including the LGB
...to of a hat with no face.
...ficer had dropped out.
...ll be your LGB Officer.
...e few students who did
...gs didn't want to be
...tive" and were only
...social gatherings. Fine,
...nge discos.
...of these discos (held in
...U back room), I heard a
...utside. In the stairwell,
...ice for heterosexual
... men were kissing.
...complained to the
...he men had been asked
...us bouncer been
...ling to the SU policy,
...the complainant to
...e had not been prop
...cause the LGB group
...ally active"
...econd year (and I was
...er, my smiley face in
..., my partner and
...oved from one hall to
... threats of gang rape
...s in our hall. Note: we
...ot them. We were
...we took the matter
...uld say goodbye to our
...equal ops.
...r stories include a
...urled downstairs by
...of a house-mate,
... her as a rival. In one
...ersity had three
...e) male rapes and
...s of women.
...st each other.
...around hall alone at
...s go to parties with
...n't know. Students
...at university is just
...s the real world.
... stop talking
...ook at facts.
...to put anyone off
...er this advice. Fight
...If there's no equal
...olicy, write and make
...But still carry a
...keep you head down
...ecked out the
...r fellow students.

I AM 38 and have been
married for four years. Our
first child, a girl, was born
three months ago — perfect
and beautiful. She died
when she was just three
days old.

Initially, the registered
cause of death was sudden
infant death syndrome or
"cot death". But then our
local hospital notified us
that her death was due to an
"overwhelming infection"
of a strain of bacteria,
Streptococcus B.

We are managing to
survive, but only just.
I wonder if anyone can
help? I have two problems.

The pragmatic
consideration first: is there
any support group for
parents who have suffered a
similar loss? Where can we
find more information
regarding this particular
bacteria? There are so many
questions I have that as yet
the hospital seems unable to
respond to.

Secondly, we are
discovering that most
people we know, in an effort
to comfort us, turn to
traditional Christian
beliefs. Without doubt we
have spiritual faith but
personally I do not accept
everything relating to
Christianity as taught to me
as a child.

People have attempted to
comfort me by saying that
my daughter and I will be
reunited in heaven, or that
she is an angel now, or even
that God only takes the
young . . . I do not find this
any comfort. I just cannot
accept a simplistic view of
heaven and hell, with us
being reunited, no doubt,
with our family dog!

Has anyone answers to
these questions?

I REMEMBER JOHN AND I "KEPT BUSY" WITH DIY PROJECTS.

I REMEMBER HEARING A WINSTON CHURCHILL QUOTE THAT WENT SOMETHING LIKE, "WHEN YOU'RE WALKING IN HELL, WALK FASTER".

ON THE DAY BILLY DIED I WAS WEARING MY DAD'S SOCKS...

JOHN'S DAD HAD DIED THE YEAR BEFORE.

I WAS GOING TO WEAR THEM ON BILLY'S OPERATION DAY BUT I THOUGHT IT WOULD BE BAD LUCK...

IF I HADN'T WORN THOSE SOCKS BILLY WOULD BE ALIVE

IF HE HADN'T WORN THOSE SOCKS BILLY WOULD STILL HAVE DIED. THEY WERE JUST SOCKS

I remember the wait while Billy was operated on...

And the impotence time imposed on us

I REMEMBER EMILY'S THOUGHTFULNESS BUT HAD FORGOTTEN OUR CONVERSATIONS.

I READ THROUGH OUR NOTES OVER AND OVER AGAIN.

THE POLICE HAVEN'T LEFT BOLLARDS IN THE STREET FOR THE FUNERAL CARS!

TYPICAL!

AFTERWARDS OUR NEXT-DOOR NEIGHBOUR KNOCKED AT THE DOOR.

A crowd outside the Rink in the 1940s

Private Lives

Last week, a mother wrote of the despair she felt when her baby daughter died at just three days old. How can she begin to come to terms with her loss?

The comfort of strangers

OUR SON died the day before we read your letter. He was two and for six months he'd had an undiagnosed respiratory illness, maybe asthma.

Unlike you, we have had no religious input and in a way it is harder. The way we grieve is not set out and we have no prescription to follow. But it is your time to do whatever makes you cope. I tell you what we tell ourselves: your baby didn't suffer in her short, sweet life and all that was possible was done. If she had suffered and then died, you would have felt empty *and* guilty. But there is nothing to say for the emptiness inside you, except that time will make the pain less acute.
Nicola Streeten
Crouch End

WE HAD also been married for four years and my wife was in her mid-thirties when our first, much tried-for baby died at birth. We witnessed the whole gamut of responses from the incredibly supportive and helpful to the sad, silly and stupid. The latter included supposedly close friends who never contacted us at the

SOME WEEKS LATER THE WORLD AROUND US RETURNED TO ITS EVERYDAY PREOCCUPATIONS ... AND WE TRIED TO AS WELL ...

I SAW WOMEN ON THEIR WAY TO WORK

AND WOMEN OFF TO THE PARK WITH CHILDREN

I DECIDED I NEEDED TO DRAMATICALLY ALTER MY APPEARANCE TO REFLECT MY CHANGED IDENTITY... SO I BOOKED IN WITH JEANA.

121

PART TWO

TIME...I KNEW IT WAS THE HEALER, BUT IN THOSE EARLY MONTHS IT WAS MY TORMENTOR... SLOW ...JEERING ...TIME ...COMBINED WITH A SEARING SENSUAL DEPRIVATION ...

THERE'S SO MUCH TOUCH INVOLVED IN
LOOKING AFTER A YOUNG CHILD....

AND YOU HAVE TO LOOK, HEAR AND
TASTE FOR THEM TOO.

MY ARMS WERE EMPTY,
MY SENSES NUMBED.

AND **TIME** WAS A
VESSEL FOR THIS ACHING
⊢————→VOID⊢——⊢

DRAWING FILLED THIS VACUUM ... ENTIRELY ... WHOLLY...

AND I DREW WHAT HAD CONSUMED MY LIFE.

I DREW MY EXPERIENCE OF PARENTING.

SOME EVENINGS I WENT TO SEE EMILY. WE HAD MET THROUGH HAVING CHILDREN AND HAD BECOME CLOSE.

MY OTHER "MUM FRIENDSHIPS" HAD POLITELY ENDED, WITH THE COMMON LINK BROKEN. WITH EMILY, THE FRIENDSHIP FOUND ANOTHER BASIS.

OH, YEAH, LOOK! I DREW THIS FOR A FRIEND

. . .

IF YOU CHANGED THE FORMAT IT WOULD MAKE A GOOD GREETING CARD. SHALL I SHOW MY PARTNER?*

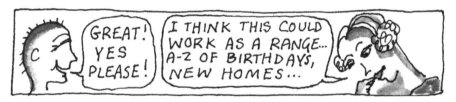

GREAT! YES PLEASE!

I THINK THIS COULD WORK AS A RANGE... A-Z OF BIRTHDAYS, NEW HOMES...

HER PARTNER THOUGHT THEY WOULDN'T SELL, BUT AGREED TO COMMISSION SIX TITLES BECAUSE EMILY LIKED THE IDEA.

LUCKILY THEY SOLD VERY VERY QUICKLY SO I COULD DRAW MORE.

*A GREETING CARD PUBLISHER

131

DRAWING ALLEVIATED MY NEED TO TALK ABOUT DEATH, BUT I STILL <u>THOUGHT</u> ABOUT IT CONSTANTLY. I GREW DEATH ANTENNAE.

FAMOUS PERSON'S BABY DIES

DO THEY FEEL LIKE ME, OR IS IT MORE PAINFUL IF YOU ARE FAMOUS?

SO AND SO'S TEENAGE SON WAS KILLED

OH, MUM, HOW AWFUL

WILL THE PARENTS FEEL LIKE ME OR IS THE PAIN GREATER IF YOUR CHILD IS OLDER?

THEN I FOUND MYSELF RANKING DEATH IN THE LINE-UP OF EMOTIONAL TRAUMA.

SO AND SO'S OFF WORK. SHE'S SEPARATED FROM HER HUSBAND

OH, MUM, THAT'S PATHETIC. NO ONE'S EVEN DIED!

OR IS THE PAIN SIMILAR?

AROUND THAT TIME, MY GRANNY, A COMMITTED HYPOCHONDRIAC, ANNOUNCED WITH DELIGHT A RECENT DIAGNOSIS.

AND DO YOU KNOW, MY DOCTOR SAID SCIATICA IS THE WORST PAIN THERE IS

OH, POOR YOU

???

THAT'S RIDICULOUS! HOW CAN A DOCTOR SAY THAT? IS THERE A UNIVERSAL HIERARCHY OF PAIN?

I HAVE HIGH-RANKING PAIN

ANYWAY... I APPOINTED MYSELF AS SOMETHING OF A DEATH EXPERT. SO WHEN MY FRIEND'S FATHER DIED I WAS TAKEN ABACK BY MY RESPONSE...

OH. I'M SORRY

SIMPLE ACKNOWLEDGEMENT CAN'T CAUSE OFFENCE ...OR IS IT TOO LITTLE?

SHOULD I SEND FLOWERS? ARE LILIES NAFF? DO I WRITE A LETTER? DO I NEED AN INVITATION TO THE FUNERAL?

DO I BUY A CARD? ...BUT THEY'RE SO INSIPID AND DULL

NEW PUPPY
BIRTHDAY
WEDD
GOOD LUCK
NEW CAR

EMILY, PLEASE CAN WE DO AN A-Z OF DEATH CARD? IT COULD BE SO FUNNY!

HMM...LET ME THINK ABOUT IT. I'M JUST NOT SURE THERE'S A MARKET

SHE'S NOT OVER THE GRIEF YET

HIS RETURN TO PART-TIME ART TEACHING IN ADULT EDUCATION WAS LESS HELPFUL...

I UNDERSTOOD THE THEORY RATHER SIMPLISTICALLY.
IN HINDSIGHT, THE LIVING OF THESE STAGES WAS LESS TIDY.

AS MONTHS WENT BY, JOHN AND I FOUND WALKING AND TALKING BECAME IMPORTANT.

MARSEILLE, FRANCE. JOHN WAS INVITED TO EXHIBIT HIS ARTWORK. I WENT WITH HIM TO HELP INSTALL THE PIECE.

ALTHOUGH I WAS STILL CONVINCED I HAD "DONE" MY STAGES OF GRIEF AND WAS THEREFORE "BETTER", MY DAILY CRYING CONTINUED.

ONE MORNING MARIE DROPPED BY WITH AN IDEA.

SUDDENLY I GOT AN "ANGER STAGE".

WE CONTINUED TO SEE OUR SEPARATE
PSYCHOLOGISTS. THIS IS WHAT THE PROCESS
HAD BEEN LIKE FOR ME...

me

psychologist

SO I STARTED TO "SEE SOMEONE" AT THE TAVISTOCK.

me

psychologist

TEN MONTHS AFTER BILLY DIED I GOT PREGNANT.

WHAT IF IT'S A **GIRL**?

WHAT IF IT'S A **BOY**?

WHAT IF WE FORGET BILLY? WHAT IF THIS BABY DIES TOO?

WHAT IF I LOVE IT MORE? WHAT IF I LOVE IT LESS? WHAT IF THIS BABY HAS HEART DEFECTS TOO?

ONCE OUR WORRIES WERE VOICED IN THIS SAFE ENVIRONMENT THEY BEGAN TO DISSIPATE.

AS WEEKS PASSED I GREW TO HATE THE TEACHING. IN THE MORNINGS JOHN WALKED WITH ME TO THE SCHOOL.

FINALLY, TIME BROUGHT US TO THE BIRTH OF OUR SECOND CHILD, SALLY.

WITH OUR NEW BABY
WE WERE "NORMAL" AGAIN.
BUT I HADN'T ANTICIPATED
HOW DIFFERENT OUR
NORMALITY WOULD HAVE
BECOME

IS THIS STILL A VASE?

IS THIS STILL A VASE?

WHICH IS NORMAL?

THE STUDIO BUILDING IS SOLD. WE'LL HAVE TO FIND SOMEWHERE ELSE

I WISH WE COULD FIND A LIVE-WORK SPACE!

YES...A NON-DOMESTIC BUILDING...I'D LOVE TO DO A CONVERSION

ME TOO. MAYBE WE COULD...IT DOESN'T HAVE TO BE IN LONDON...

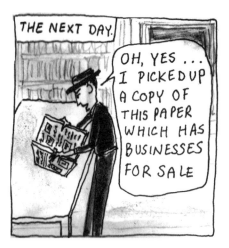

THE NEXT DAY.

OH, YES... I PICKED UP A COPY OF THIS PAPER WHICH HAS BUSINESSES FOR SALE

LOOK AN EMPTY PUB. THAT WOULD BE GOOD

EXCEPT IT'S ON THE INTERSECTION OF TWO MOTORWAYS

OOH, A SUB POST OFFICE IN WALES IS CHEAP

THIS LOOKS INTERESTING... A METHODIST CHAPEL IN LINCOLNSHIRE

MEMORIES

OF

BILLY

In Memoriam

BILLY Edwin Plowman **STREETEN**
3 July 1993 - 19 September 1995
Billy boy, Billy boy, playing in his den,
Billy boy, Billy boy, with his band of friends,
Loved by his mum, loved by his dad,
Billy boy, Billy boy.

When Billy was alive, we made up
a little song to the Robin Hood tune.
At his funeral we invited everyone to
sing along... Every year since, John has
put an IN MEMORIAM in the newspaper.
This year there was a line left out...

In Memoriam

BILLY Edwin Plowman **STREETEN**
Billy boy, Billy boy, playing in his den,
Billy boy, Billy boy, with his band of friends,
Loved by his mum, loved by his dad,
Billy boy, Billy boy.

I FEEL SO GUILTY. I WAS SO BUSY I DIDN'T CHECK IT WAS OK

IT'S FINE! IT DOESN'T MEAN WE'VE STOPPED REMEMBERING BILLY

Billy Edwin Plowman Streeten

3 July 1993 — 19 September 1995

30 May 95

AND EVERY DAY HE DREW WITH INCREASING CONFIDENCE...
LITTLE REPETITIVE STUDIES OF "NEE NARS".

THIS WAS BILLY'S FAVOURITE BOOK...

AS SOON AS BILLY HAD LEARNT TO WALK CONFIDENTLY, HE INSISTED ON "DRIVING".

...STOPPING OFF FOR A DRINK BREAK NOW AND THEN...

...AT HOME HE'D SPEND TIME PLAYING WITH HIS TOY CAR COLLECTION.

BILLY "HELPED" ME PLANT SEEDS IN THE GARDEN.

THREE SUNFLOWERS GREW, TALL AND BOLD.

THE DAY BEFORE BILLY'S OPERATION, I CUT THEM DOWN AND TOOK THEM INTO THE HOSPITAL.

The following day ...

AFTERWORD

I HAD SIGNED UP TO DO A MASTER'S DEGREE, FOR WHICH I WOULD EMBARK ON A GRAPHIC NOVEL. AN EARLY ASSIGNMENT WAS TO PRESENT OUR PROPOSALS TO THE CLASS.

THE GENDER BALANCE IN THE GRAPHIC NOVEL IN THE U.K, IN THE 21ST CENTURY

BLA BLA BLA HISTORY OF COMICS

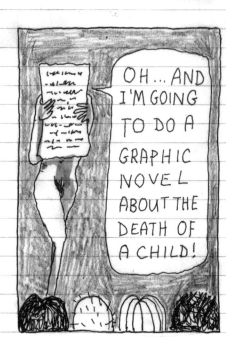

OH... AND I'M GOING TO DO A GRAPHIC NOVEL ABOUT THE DEATH OF A CHILD!

I SAID A CHILD... OF COURSE I MEANT MY CHILD.

LUCKILY THERE WAS AN OPPORTUNITY FOR CRITICAL FEEDBACK.

I REALISED MY NARRATIVE HAD BEGUN AND THAT I HAD NO EASY TASK AHEAD.

I WAS ALLOCATED A PERSONAL TUTOR.

MEANWHILE, I ATTENDED SOME PUBLIC TALKS ABOUT "THE GRAPHIC NOVEL".

WHERE ARE THE WOMEN?

RUDE

OH, BE QUIET AND READ FOUCAULT

TOTALLY IRRELEVANT

HUH, FEMINIST

HA HA, BRILLIANT

DYKE

I GOT CHATTING TO AN ARTIST WHO'D ALSO BEEN IN THE AUDIENCE.

WOULDN'T IT BE GREAT TO HAVE A SORT OF CLUB WHERE WE COULD TALK ABOUT THE WORKS WE LIKE... MORE DOMESTIC THAN SUPERHEROES

NOT EXCLUSIVELY FOR WOMEN, BUT WHERE WOMEN ARE COMFORTABLE

CAKE

WE COULD INVITE PEOPLE WE THINK ARE GREAT TO TALK ABOUT THEIR WORK.

LAYDEEZ DO COMICS WAS SET UP IN 2009.

WE SOLD COPIES OF OUR COMIC-MAG
TO FAMILY, FRIENDS AND SUBSCRIBERS.

EACH ISSUE INCLUDED A CHAPTER
OF "MY GRAPHIC NOVEL".

ACKNOWLEDGEMENTS

This book is about a time when I felt emotions with an extremity not experienced before or since, and here it is condensed into a story. The three-and-a-half years in the making has not been a sad experience for me, but a creatively rewarding and satisfying time. I am indebted to many people for their roles, both in the original unfolding and in the telling of it in this form. I thank them all, especially our families and friends.

Most importantly, I thank my soul mate and husband, John Plauman and our lovely daughter, Sally Plauman, who restored true happiness into our lives again. John, I thank for his collaborative approach to life with me. Sally, I thank for the idea and eagerness to start Liquorice and for the laughs we have had working on it together. A special mention to Holly, the dog, a key player in Liquorice and our lives! I thank all the essential supporters of Liquorice, who have subscribed and offered feedback. This group of people became my first readers and provided a vital testing of material.

My research into comics and the graphic novel has introduced me to a world of interesting and inspiring people. In particular, I thank Sarah Lightman, artist, curator and academic, with whom I never run out of things to talk and laugh about. This project would not have come to fruition without her friendship and the work we have done together, principally setting up Laydeez do Comics, in 2009. Thank you to all who have attended, as presenters, bloggers and audience.

Finally, I thank the team at Myriad Editions, who have been such a delight to work with. Especially Corinne Pearlman, who has given so much time and guidance to shaping the work with me from the outset.

Nicola Streeten, 2011

MORE FROM MYRIAD EDITIONS